ELIZABETH SHELTON

Brush Like A Boss

The Ultimate Guide To Caring For The Teeth You Want To Keep

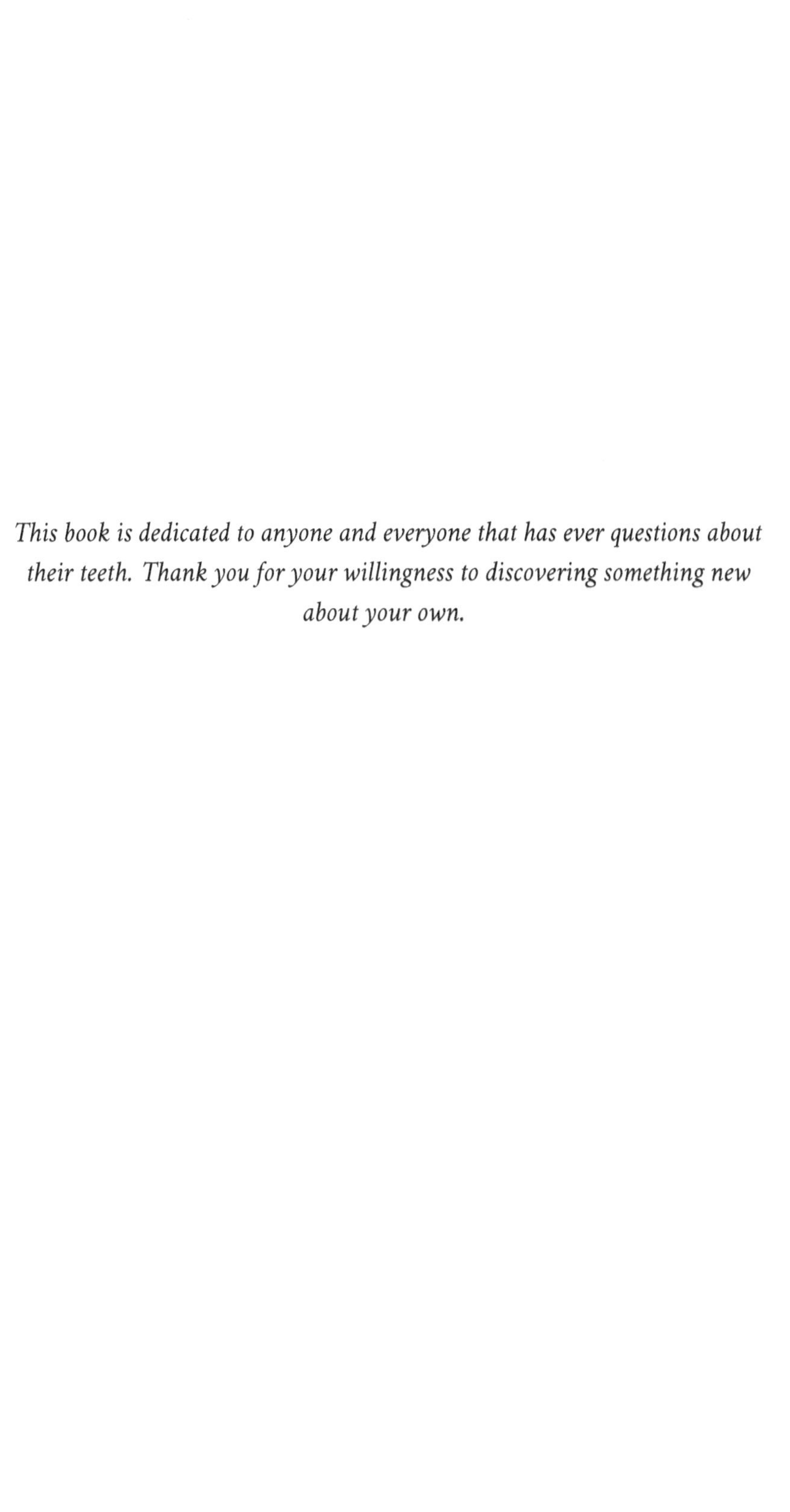

This book is dedicated to anyone and everyone that has ever questions about their teeth. Thank you for your willingness to discovering something new about your own.

Contents

1

Introduction to Brush Like A Boss

Welcome to Brush Like A Boss: The Ultimate Guide to Caring For The Teeth You Want To Keep! My name is Elizabeth Shelton; I am so excited to be writing this book! This book will help guide us in keeping our oral hygiene in order to keep the teeth we want. Whether it be the first tooth, the last tooth or somewhere in between (even the gums), this book will help guide you in the right direction!

Furthermore, I am very passionate about this book because there is so much to know about our teeth and gums and how they connect to the body as a whole! Many do not know this, but the gateway to our overall health lies in how we care for our teeth and gums! They are connected to a lot of the health concerns in society nowadays IE: diabetes, high blood pressure, high cholesterol, stress, etc!

A little about me, like previously mentioned above, my name is Elizabeth Shelton. I have been a part of the dental field for over 13 years and counting. Although I wanted to continue my education and become a dentist and even specialize in a specific field of dentistry, life took me on a different route. We often think our lives will take us one way, but it will continue to lead us until our destination! To this day, I am very passionate about dentistry and am excited to share all that I have learned on this journey thus far! Perhaps, I will write another book focusing on specific dental specialties and why each one is just as important as the next one.

For now, this book will focus on oral hygiene and how to care for, like the title states, the teeth you want to keep! Now, this book will not give every specific detail regarding our teeth, like the anatomy and life span of each tooth. It will however give you the reassurance of why we brush, floss, rinse, repeat and of course how to help assure you maximize the time you have left with the teeth and gums you have!

You can read this book cover to cover, if you choose, or you can pick it up and turn to a specific chapter to help guide you in that area of questioning. Also, what I love about this book is that it is user friendly for all ages! In other words, it is written as simply as possible, any age can read and gain to understand something from it!

All this being said, I should mention to be advised that this book is intended to be a reference guide and should not be used as a medical manual in diagnosing any sorts of overall health or oral concerns. This book is to help you make an informed decision on how to care for your teeth and gums. Should you have extensive health concerns, I strongly advise you to seek medical and dental professional care. Resources will be sited at the end and throughout the book to help clarify and questions.

Without further ado, if you are ready to dive into a world of 'ahh, I see', let's get started!

2

What is oral health care and why is it important?

According to the definition given by the World Health Organization, "Oral health is the state of the mouth, teeth and orofacial structures that enables individuals to perform essential functions such as eating, breathing and speaking, and encompasses psychosocial dimensions such as self-confidence, well-being and the ability to socialize and work without pain, discomfort and embarrassment. Oral health varies over the life course from early life to old age, is integral to general health and supports individuals in participating in society and achieving their potential." https://www.who.int/health-topics/oral-health#tab=tab_1

In simple terms, oral health is the art keeping of your teeth and gums clean by staying disease free, cavity free and pain free in order to continue doing the things you love to do. Whether it be the elderly stage where we just have our gums to the early stages of life with our baby teeth (primary teeth). To the between stages of life with our adult teeth (permanent teeth) you care for the teeth and gums you want to keep, simple as that!

Now, I won't go on as to tell you when to expect each stage, however, the importance of caring for our oral health at each step is vital to our general health as a whole! Come with me as we dive into this sensitive matter that is indeed considered taboo.

3

When should I visit the dentist?

As soon as you feel a 'bump' or see a white, raised area in the baby's mouth. Most of the time, when this happens, chances are the baby is going to get a new tooth soon! As most experienced parents will know, there is a tell-tale sign when this is happening (heightened fussiness, drooling and even chewing on anything and everything!), but not all know it is highly recommended to take the child to see the dentist. Some may think, 'meh, it's just a tooth, all is well' but in fact this is the best time to establish patient care!

Actually, your dentist will be able to help inform you whether or not it is actually a tooth beginning to erupt or something that may be a little more concerning (like thrush or even a bone spicule). This will help you get ahead of the care for your infant and avoid any major concerns you may have later down the road.

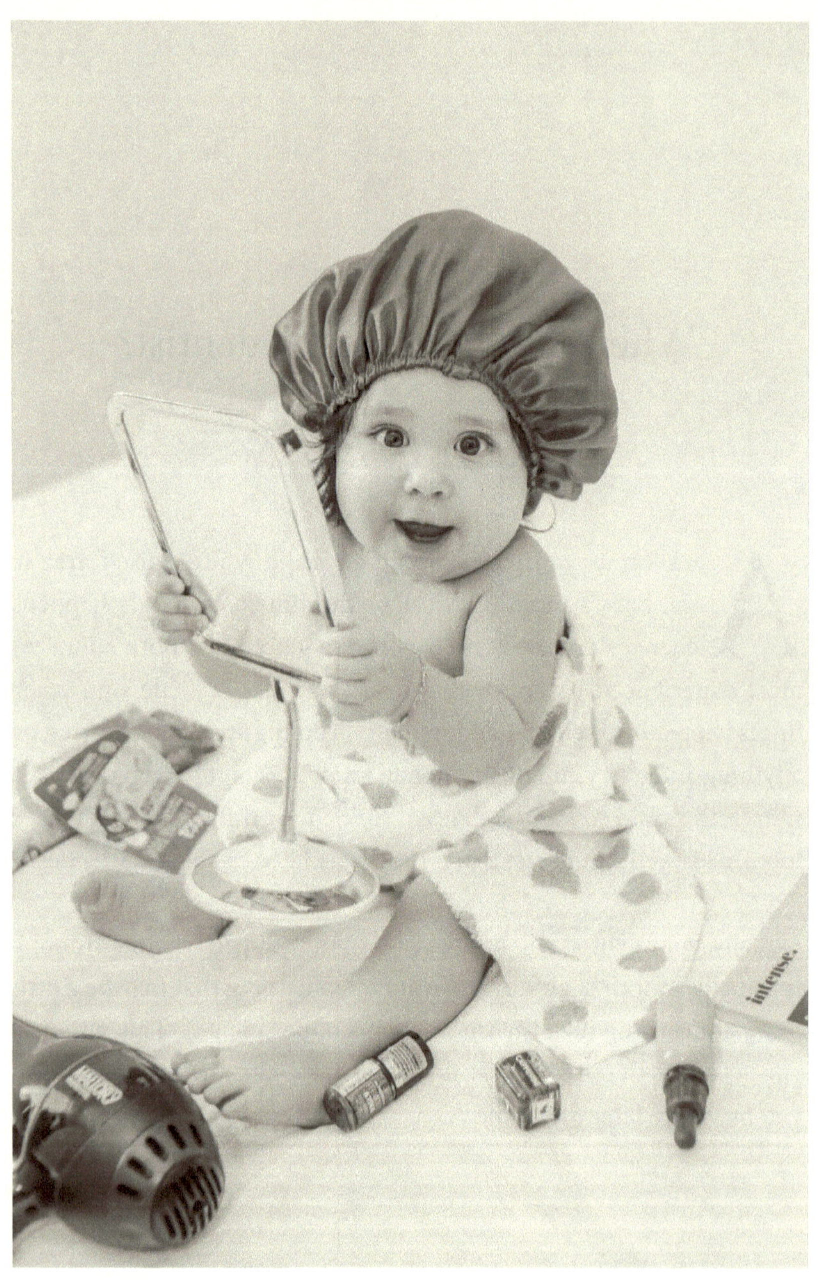

This also helps establish care from the start! Not to bash on anyone who is afraid of the dentist, but I have seen my share of dental anxiety in all ages. I do not care how experienced of a patient you may be or if you're in the dental field, DENTAL ANXIETY is normal, even for the experienced patient and your dental team! It's different when you are the one in the chair. However, this can be honed and better treated and cared for in the chair when you are seen for regular checkups and treatment from childhood.

Now this does not excuse all the dental trauma stories, because there are cases where they could have been due to bedside manner (how you are treated at the dental office) but that's another book in itself. All in all, establishing care from the start will help reduce the anxiety and gain the experience needed to help kick that and avoid bad experiences at the dental office that make patients fearful of ever returning until it's too late to save that tooth you wanted to keep! Also key-worthy, if you do have a bad experience at one dental office, this does not mean you won't find an office that won't deliver the treatment you deserve! We, as a dental profession, care and want to help you the best way we can and know. You just have to trust we are here to help!

4

Taking care of the gums also known as the gingiva

I only have my gums, how is that important? Great question! Whether it's just your gums or you have little to no teeth, the best oral hygiene is caring for your gums!

Our gums tend to 'change form' as we age. Whether it be a young child, bone structure growing and forming, to the elderly and in between, decreased bone structure, our gums will increase or decrease with the amount of bone available. The gums act as a 'protect-ant layer' to the underlying bone structure and can either be bulky and healthy or minimal and thin sitting on top of the bone (jaw structure). Either way, the gums (or in dental terminology gingiva), is vital to our overall health.

In order to keep the gums healthy, believe it or not, you do have to maintain care of them! The best way to do so is in fact with a sterile (clean) towel or a 'gum brush'.

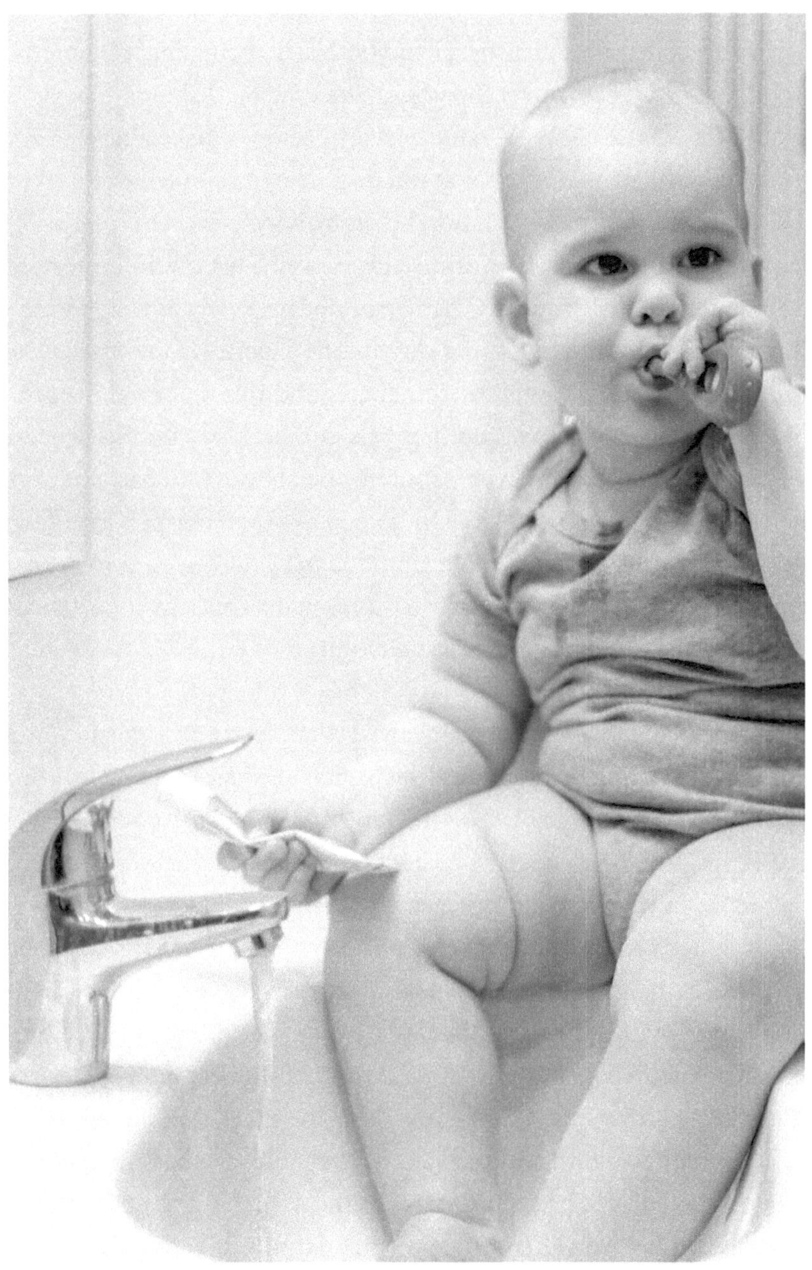

Gum brushes are very light weight and fit right over the finger to act as a normal toothbrush. Then you brush, your finger being the toothbrush! Of course, toothpaste can be used but I should warn you, not all toothpaste tastes the same to every person. What could be minty fresh to you can in fact be spicy and disgusting to someone else (even babies). Now if using a clean towel (I really hope you are), please make absolutely sure you are not using a dry towel! This is very important as you may actually hurt the baby and not help. My advice, wet the towel with lukewarm water, and ring out the majority of the water. Like the finger brush, you will use one finger and run the towel over the gums with light pressure. Toothpaste is not necessary for this process although can be used with precautions said above. Your baby may cry but you also know their cries. Once you have used one portion of the towel to 'brush' the gums, move onto the next clean area of the towel and repeat your steps. You can do this as many times as you'd like or until you feel the gums are nice and clean!

Regardless if there are no teeth involved when finger brushing or towel brushing, keeping the gums healthy is vital in order to maintain your overall health (baby or not). Now this goes to say you may or may not get push back from the person when doing so, especially a baby! My advice, lay them in your lap and proceed to brush upside down! They will indeed kick and scream at times but it is very important you continue to brush as many teeth as you can until you feel you've brushed all areas of the mouth or if the screaming is excessive. The more you introduce this method to them, the greater the experience is next time you 'brush' their gums. Before you know it, brushing their teeth (once they arrive) will become second nature to them. They may even enjoy doing so themselves and can brush their own teeth. With this, my advice would be to brush for them first then let them do it so you know all areas are being cared for. This also helps them build their cognitive skills.

5

My teeth and what they do for me

Okay so now we all know what teeth are but for those who do not know, it's the hard things inside our mouths that come out of the gums and help us chew our food so we can digest things better and live. Not trying to be funny, maybe a little sarcastic, but it's the simplest way I can explain what our teeth are and what they do for us. Now the benefits of having teeth, especially ALL of your teeth, is in fact, what I stated earlier. They help us chew our food. Don't quote me, but I'm almost certain I've read somewhere that you're technically supposed to chew your food 60-90 times prior to swallowing.

According to google, you're supposed to chew your food 30-40 times before swallowing, depending on how hard the item is. For softer foods, 5-10 times before swallowing. It also states that this helps to increase the amount of nutrients you get out of your food. Apparently it helps with weight control too.

Now some of you reading may or may not have all your teeth. Kudos to you if you do, but if you don't I'm sure eating can be difficult at times.

For those who cannot relate, imagine losing a tooth.

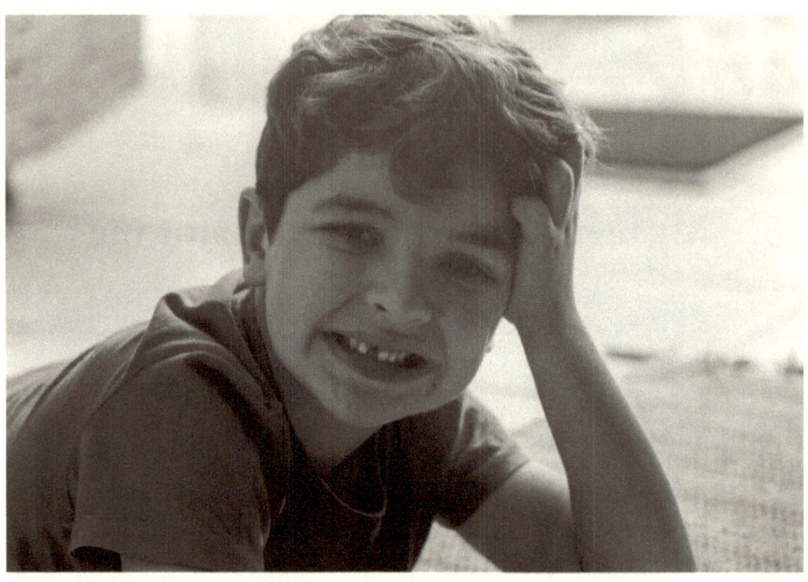

Now imagine eating a carrot and the tooth you lost is on the same side you favor chewing. You're eating and bam as you're eating, a piece of the carrot jabs you right in the gum in that empty space. Now imagine having this happen with multiple areas with missing teeth. Don't feel good right?

Keep them as long as you can, you'll regret it when you lose one. For those who have missing teeth, visit your dentist for replacement options should you decide to gain the chance to enjoy food better. One thing I cannot stress enough to anyone and everyone. When replacing the tooth, please understand the replacement tooth will not be the same nor will it ever be your tooth you lost. It is what it actually is, a replacement tooth.

Some people end up falling in love with the replacement tooth (teeth, option). Some, unfortunately, do not. If you do not like it, and have the finances to do so, go to your dentist and see if there are any other options for you. But with all due respect, some of us will never be satisfied with the replacement option because we have our hopes set on it functioning and maybe even cosmetically looking like the tooth you lost, your natural tooth/teeth. This is why I say to not set your hopes so high in having that functionality back. A replacement tooth is nothing like the natural tooth you were born with. Thus the name. Don't set yourself up with that type of frustration. You'll end up disappointed every time. Go in with an open mind, really sit back, acknowledge and understand the replacement tooth is your choice. At the end of the day, you decide whether or not you want that chance to eat better than you have since losing the tooth.

6

Plaque, gum disease and other oral health concerns

If you run your tongue over your teeth after a meal, you'll feel like something is lying between your tongue and the smoothness of your teeth. That barrier you feel is plaque. It's a sticky, color-less film on your teeth after you eat. How much longer? Not too sure, everyone is different and every food is different, just know that film you feel, should not stay on your teeth for long.

In fact, plaque is actually the gateway to all the other oral health concerns we gain if we do not care for our teeth properly. If I were speaking with a child, I would explain plaque as being a sugar bug. If the sugar bug stays on our teeth too long it starts eating at our teeth making holes where they like to stay and make a home. These holes are usually described as decay or caries (cavities) in the dental terminology. If holes get too big, we tend to have pain follow. Sometimes this pain can be taken care of and the tooth can be saved by our dentist and the team.

Other times, the pain and damage is too much and the sugar bugs have done so much damage, the only way to get you out of the pain is to in fact remove the tooth and discuss replacement options. Usually our gums can help tell us whether there could be something else happening in our mouths that to the naked eye can't see.

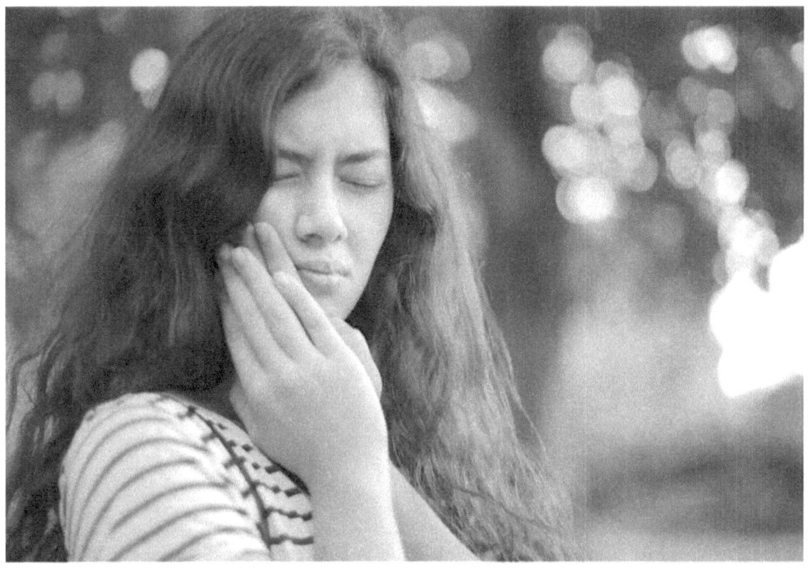

Gum disease also known as periodontal disease is in fact a real thing. This disease can indeed affect not only the gums but the bone lying underneath the gums as well as the teeth growing out of them. Picture a plant growing out of the ground. If the soil is not maintained and of course watered regularly, the plant will struggle to survive. This is quite the same as our gums. If we are not properly supporting the gums, they will bleed and most times look swollen. You will experience pain when eating, drinking and even brushing. Most times, bad breath is associated with this and even worse, the gum can indeed separate from the teeth and supporting bone and will in fact cause the tooth to become loose and fall out.

There are indeed several other diseases including edentulism, Noma and even oral cancer, but again as mentioned, I'm not here to explain nor scare anyone with these cases. Should you decide to do your own research on these and other extensive diseases that may occur, I have included a link to the World Health Organization. https://www.who.int/news-room/fact-sheets/detail/oral-health

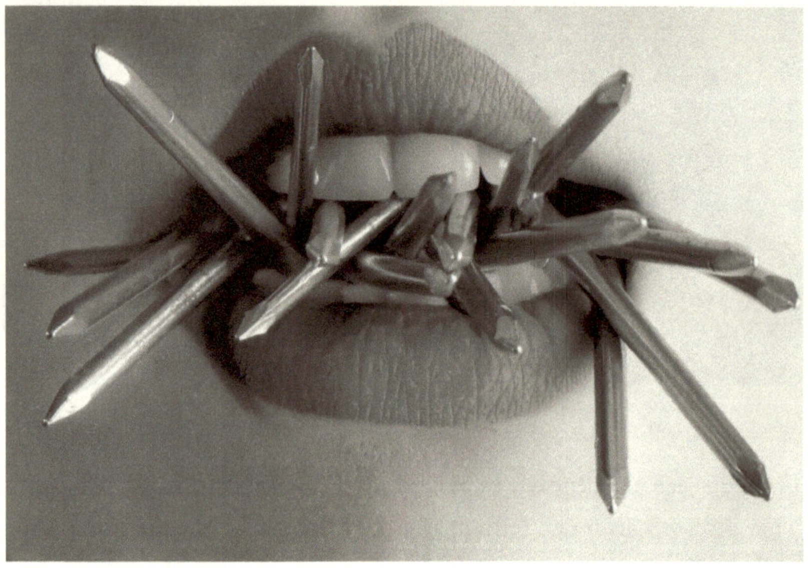

Now that I've mentioned all of the above, you are probably saying to yourself, 'YES, I do have bleeding of my gums!' or 'Yes, my gums are swollen and sometimes I do feel a film on my teeth!' Yes, to it all! But how do we fix the problems!? Well for starters, how we take care of our teeth and gums is top priority! Let's move along and I'll help guide you with oral hygiene.

7

Brushing: the ins, outs and everything between

Alright, we've got to the section where everyone is wondering about brushing habits and am I doing this right? Well first off, brushing is going to be different for everyone because, well, we all have different teeth. Whether it be one tooth or all teeth, baby teeth or grown up teeth and even no teeth and all gums, the care you show your gums and teeth will definitely reflect in your health. All this to say, please TAKE CARE OF YOUR THEM BOTH. Or at the very least, take care of the ones you want to keep.

I have been in the dental field for over a decade and each dental provider I have conversed with has had a different brushing technique. Onc thing is for certain, all have uniformly agreed brushing your teeth and gums right before bed time is crucial. We are constantly eating and drinking and introducing different things into our mouths all day everyday. The last thing you want to do is let the 'sugar bugs' sit overnight and make a bigger home on your teeth.

The most effective way of brushing is in fact focusing the toothbrush at an angle towards the gums in circular motions at the base of the tooth and gums. In other words, brush where the gum and teeth meet. I myself have always been told brushing up and down, side to side and circular motions are most effective. But realistically, whatever motion you decide to brush in, the fact that you're brushing is indeed something to take into consideration. Be proud of that and then revise and perfect. Brushing just the top part of the teeth and not by the gums, leaves the sugar bugs to attack the root and gums and enter the blood system where again, disease can happen and affect everywhere else in the body.

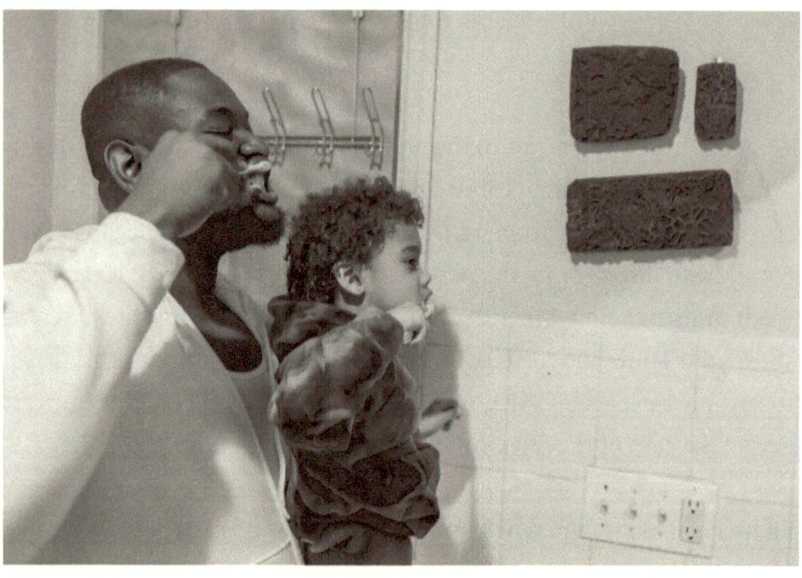

Now this goes to say the reason we brush is not because we want pearly white teeth (although most of us do). It's because we want to be healthy at least to have the best chance at being healthy. It hurts to brush, my gums bleed when I brush, I can't do this. Well, what is it we were always told? Practice makes perfect? If you want to succeed, try, try again?

Rome wasn't built overnight? Excuses are just that, excuses. YES, it may hurt at first, YES it may bleed for a bit. YES, you may even want to give up. I'm here to tell you the reality of all your fears of brushing is in fact true. BUT, this too shall pass and will only get better with time. Keep brushing, I guarantee you, the sensitivity will be less with each time you do.

Now the amount of time. There has always been controversy with how long we should brush. I've heard one minute, I've heard two minutes. I've even heard dental providers say they brush less than that, believe it or not. I've come to terms for my own personal brushing habits, 1-3 minutes. One thing is for certain, DO NOT forget the back of your last teeth! Keep this in mind, only brush the ones you want to keep. Simple as that, if you don't want them, then let it be.

Should I buy an electric toothbrush or stick with the toothbrushes the dentist always gives me (manual toothbrush)? My answer, whichever you feel most comfortable with. I have both. I use the electric toothbrush at home and have a manual I carry with me throughout the day. Some people feel they do just fine with the manual toothbrush and don't need the electric toothbrush. I like them both to be completely transparent. Your dental team should be truthful when you go for your routine checkups and tell you whether or not you should stick with the manual toothbrush or elevate your brushing game to an electric toothbrush. The benefits of having the electric toothbrush is the fact that it does all the work for you. You just have to move the toothbrush around the mouth. Whereas with a manual toothbrush you're choosing the motion you'd like the brush to go as well as moving it around the mouth. Like I said before, whichever you decide, just make sure you focus on brushing where the teeth and gums meet and don't forget the backside of the last tooth in each section of the mouth.

8

What about flossing and mouthwash?

Along with brushing, the habits of flossing and using mouthwash are definitely as important. Flossing helps with making sure sugar bugs that like to hide between our teeth, stay out! Mouthwash helps 'kill 99% of germs' or whatever the slogans usually say. But on a serious note, mouthwash does in fact help kill that bad breath feeling and is that extra care to our oral hygiene.

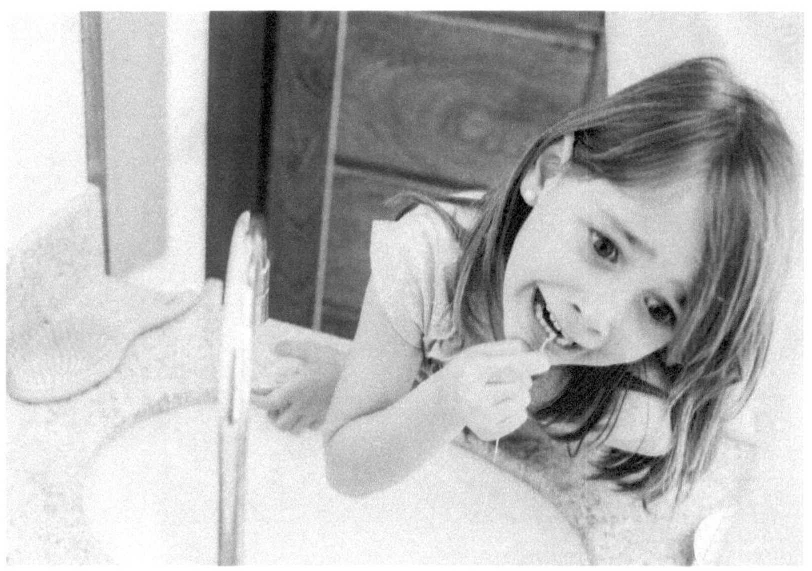

There have been several ways to floss that have been developed over the years. So you don't have to stick to the traditional string if it's too complicated to make the 'C' shape and continue along until done. Soft picks, inter-dental floss, super-floss just to name a few. All are great, you just have to decide which works for you and just like a habit we want to keep, make it a part of your daily routine. Start with one to two days out of the week to contribute flossing. Once you feel comfortable with remembering to floss on those specific days, the next week add another day making it three times a week you are flossing. Once comfortable again, continue adding another day. Eventually you'll be flossing everyday! But don't forget, floss the back of the last tooth on all sides of the mouth, we want to keep those teeth!

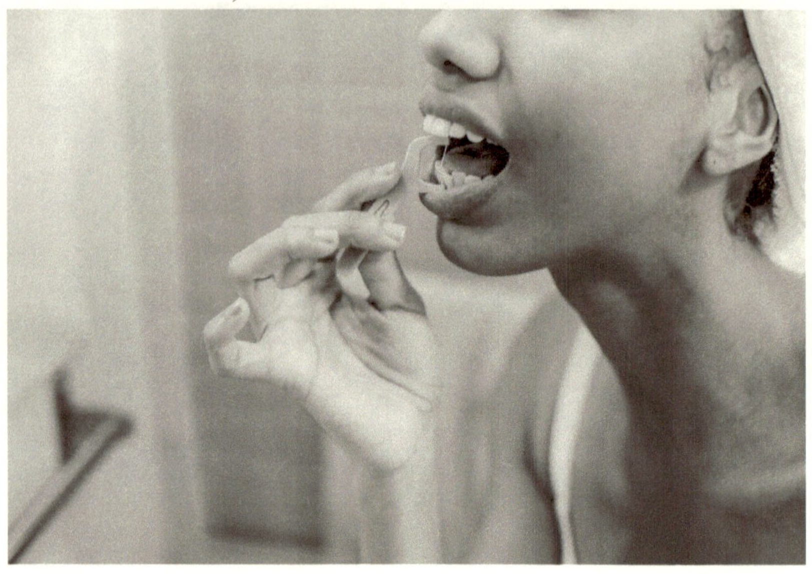

I've always had this controversial question come up in my years of dentistry. "Should I brush, floss, then use mouthwash? Or should I floss, brush then use mouthwash? Does it matter?" Yes, exactly. Does it really matter? The fact that you're actually taking the time to do all three is what matters most! Let me do you one better, how about adding water-piking to your routine?! Yes, waterpik and no, it's not the same as mouth wash and definitely does not replace flossing. There is also mouthwash out there that changes the plaque a different color and will show you where you need to focus on brushing! Of course it's more geared to kids but hey, every so often I'll use it just to see if I'm doing what I'm preaching.

I'll admit, sometimes I get lazy, that's a lot to add to a routine on the daily. Sometimes I'll even add mouthwash to my waterpik and tell myself I've done both. Ha! Way to psych the mind out right. But truth be told, water-piking helps blast out any of those unwanted and stubborn sugar bugs that stick around when simple flossing can't reach them. Again, doesn't replace but actually reinforces your oral hygiene.

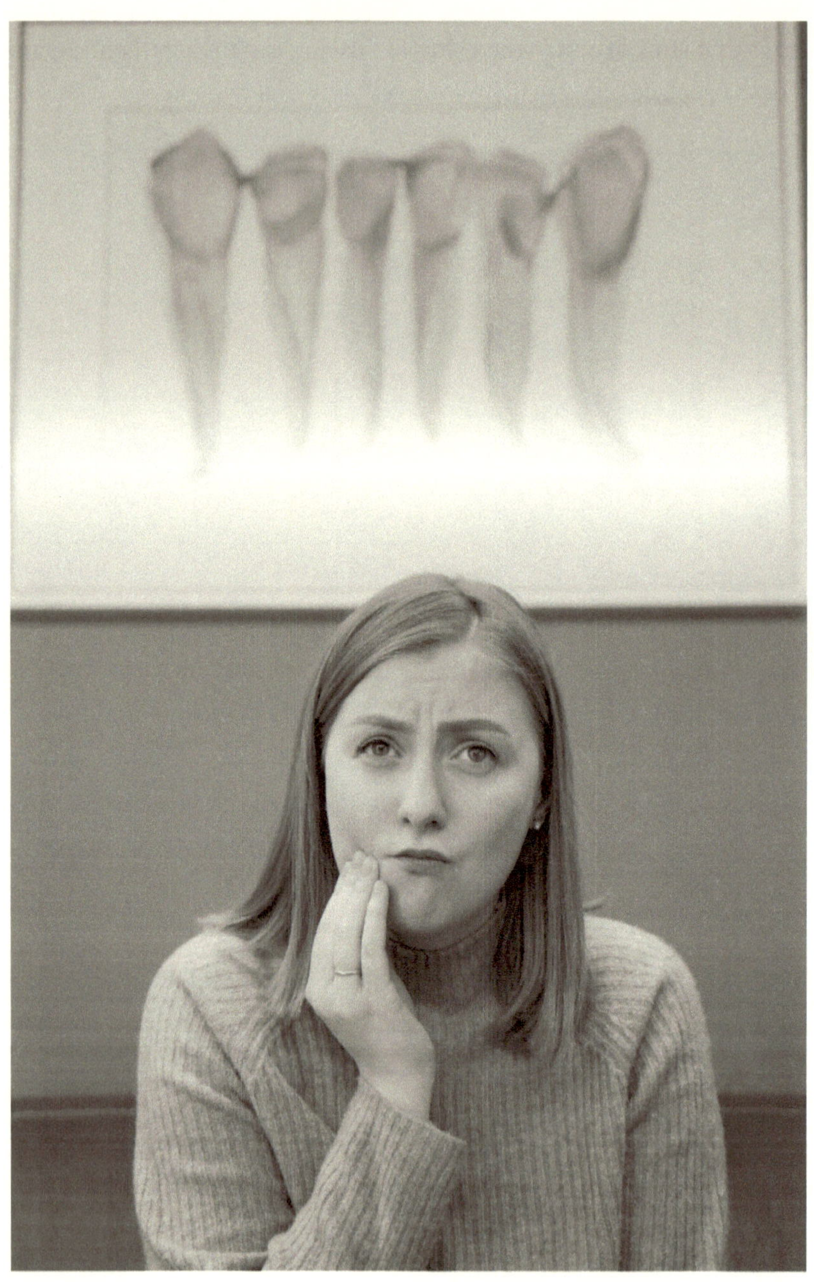

It hurts, it's uncomfortable, I don't like it, blah blah blah. Yeah but doing the uncomfortable will one day become such a habit you'll reminisce on the days you actually thought it was painful and be so proud of yourself and how far you've come with keeping up with your oral hygiene. Keep going, you've got nothing to lose, oh wait, I guess you do, your teeth and gums should you choose not to take care of them. Just have a conversation with someone who lost their teeth, if they're brave enough, they'll share their why's and do's and don't s. SO you choose, do you want to brush, floss, rinse and repeat, give up a few minutes of your time a day for a lifetime of keeping and enjoying all the benefits of having your teeth and gums or do you want to leave it as is and see what happens down the road? You decide.

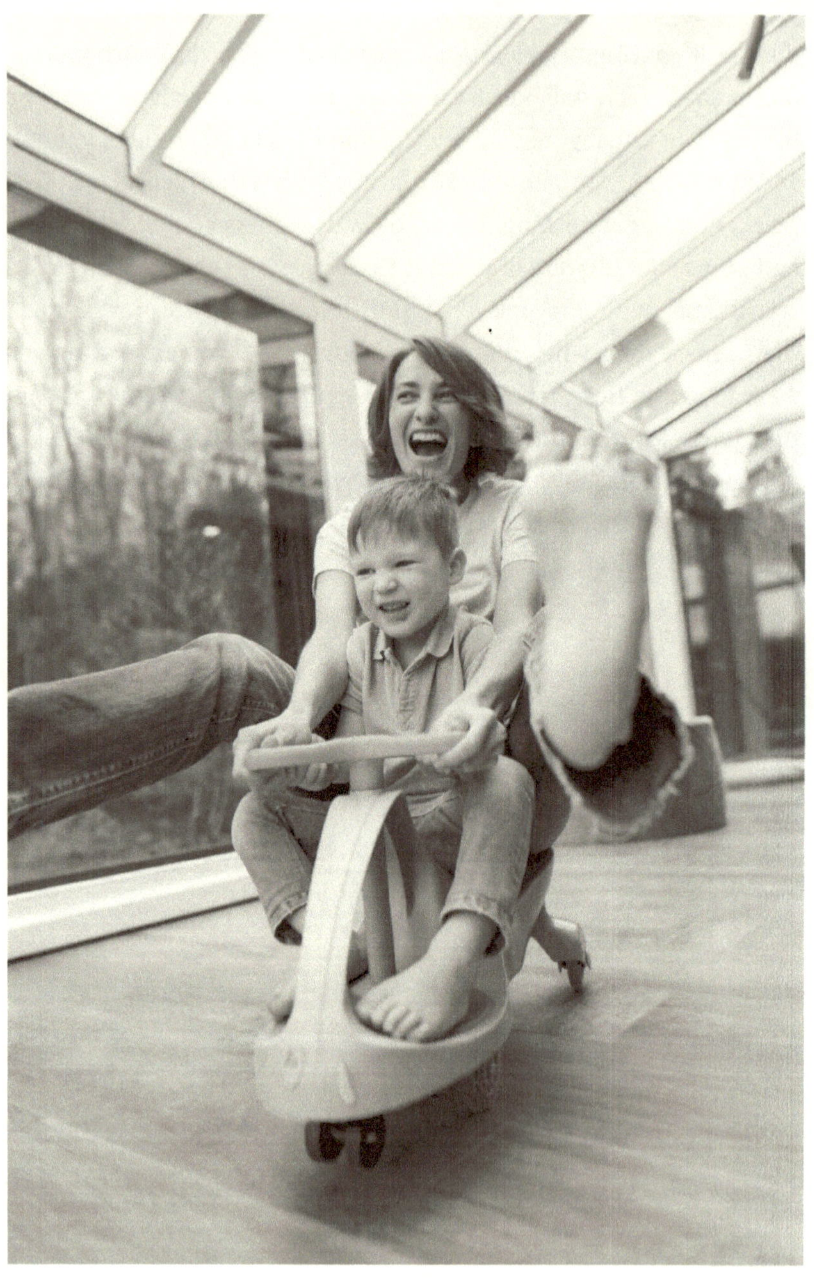

9

Should I visit the dentist or not?

Um, yes! Don't wait till the last minute when you're screaming and crying in agony because your tooth hurts and you haven't slept and you've done everything and nothing is helping. I will always say, go to your dentist! Whether it be for a regular check up or for an emergency visit, or to say hi, whatever the case may be. Go to your dentist!

Find an office that of course, takes your insurance or fits within your budget. Most places will advertise and even inform you of their prices before helping you schedule. Call, explain your case and they'll help guide you in the right direction. It's up to you to decide and of course show up to your visit. If you like the office, great, discuss the treatment plan, make sure all of your questions are answered, get a second opinion if need be, but do not let your dental care sit in the back seat of your life.

Sometimes we get patients that are truly traumatized from past experiences of being in the dental chair. That is okay! Truly. It happens, and we are in no position to judge you. Our job is to help you face your fears and get the help you need so you can continue on with your life. If you feel an office is not the right fit for you, I'm sure there are plenty of other offices that are willing to help make sure your visit is comfortable. Just take the leap, continue as much as you possibly can with your visit and reschedule if you need to but at least you showed and pushed through til you couldn't any longer.

If you're a kid, or a parent taking a child in, please understand that wanting to be in the dental operatory while working on your child in fact heightens the traumatic experience for them. I'm sorry I had to say it but you thinking you're helping in the room by reassuring your child everything is okay, is not helping! I repeat, that does not help. In fact, it makes things worse. Kids tend to act completely differently in the chair when parents are there. It's great to have you in the room at the beginning of the appointment or even there til about 4 yrs old but after that, they almost always listen and do way better when the parent is in the waiting room. We are professionals, and as professionals, we have ways in assuring your child's comfort. If it's too much for someone to handle, just like adults, we stop, reschedule and try a different route next time. What will not help is a hovering parent saying it's okay, you can continue or telling the child to stop and they're almost done, etc, etc. This in fact leads to traumatic experiences that turn to full blown anxious adult patients. As a part of your dental team, please help us, help you by cooperating with the team. It will help both the child and parent in the long run.

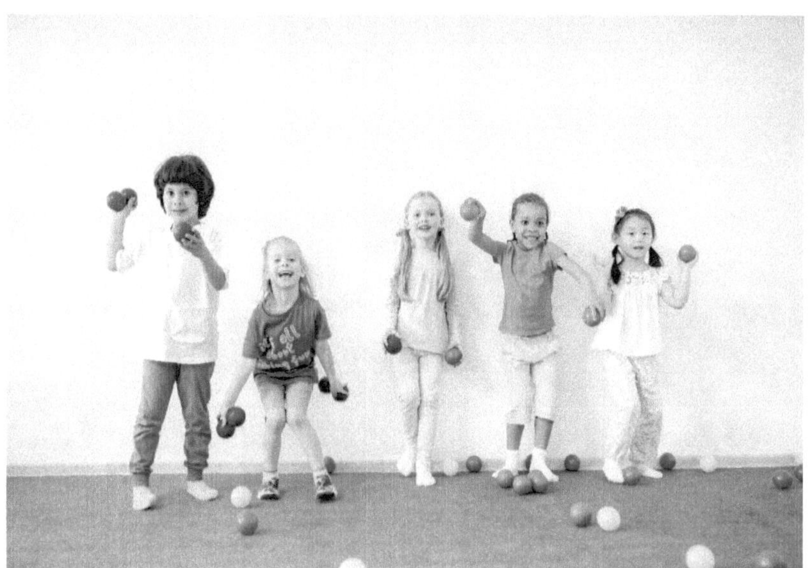

Like mentioned before, the best way to avoid traumatic adulthood experiences is in fact bringing the child in as soon as you feel the first signs of having a tooth. The more you or your child come into the office for your routine check up and cleanings, whether it be 3-4 months or even 6-months between, the better chance your dental office can get ahead of any questionable areas of the mouth. The higher chance of saving your teeth!

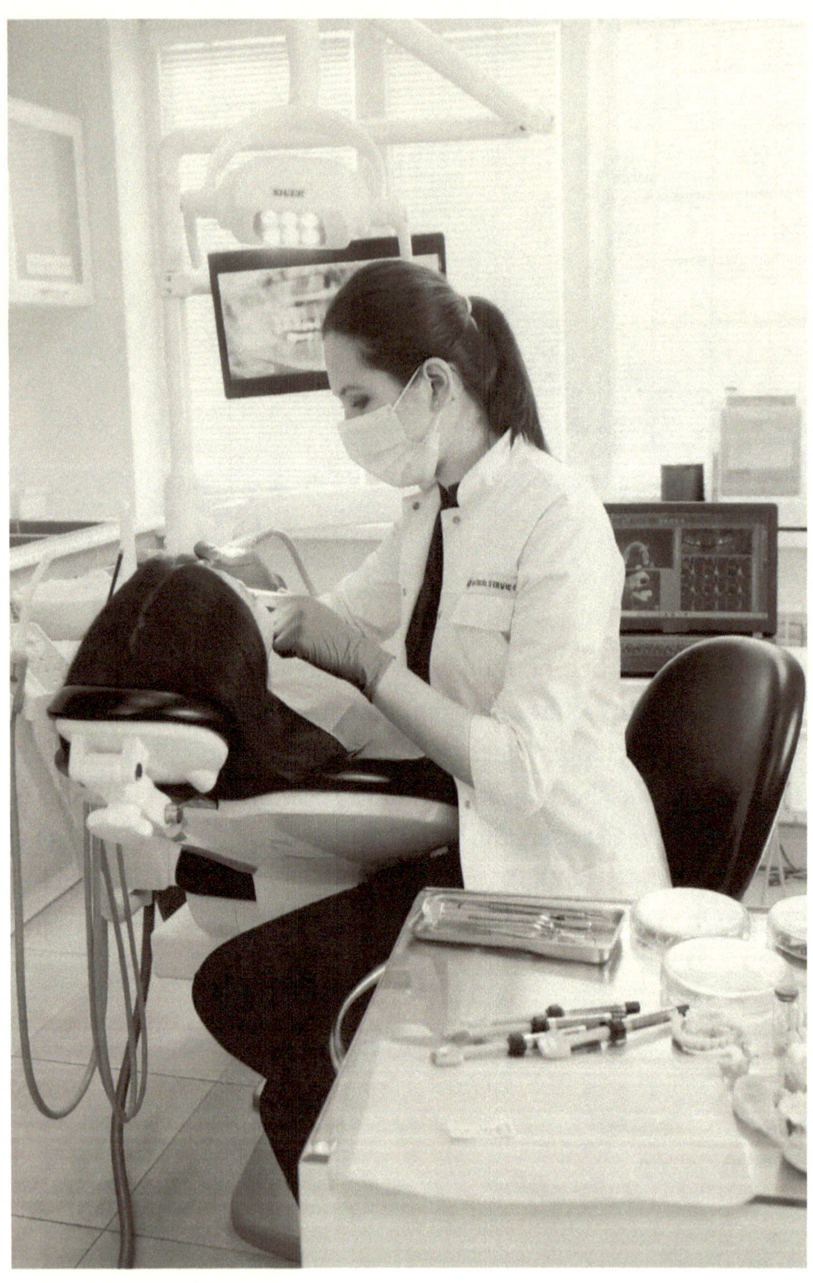

So please, come in and visit your nearest and most trustworthy dental office to you! They'll be able to answer any questions you have whether it be fluoride applications, sealant protect-ants and even restorative questions like what's a filling to the best type of floss and more. Make an appointment and actually commit to going in with an open mind. You have all the knowledge to gain about your own teeth.

10

What happens if I don't take care of my teeth?

Well the simple and probably sarcastic answer, you lose them of course. The not so sarcastic answer and probably more lengthy, did not need to say all that answer is pain. Pain, pain and more pain that probably has already started with rotting, discoloration, decalcification, halitosis, pretty much sugar bugs eating everything and anything it can. Then leads to a dental visit. That worst case scenario ends with you losing your essential tooth or you paying an unexpected cost to save your essential tooth.

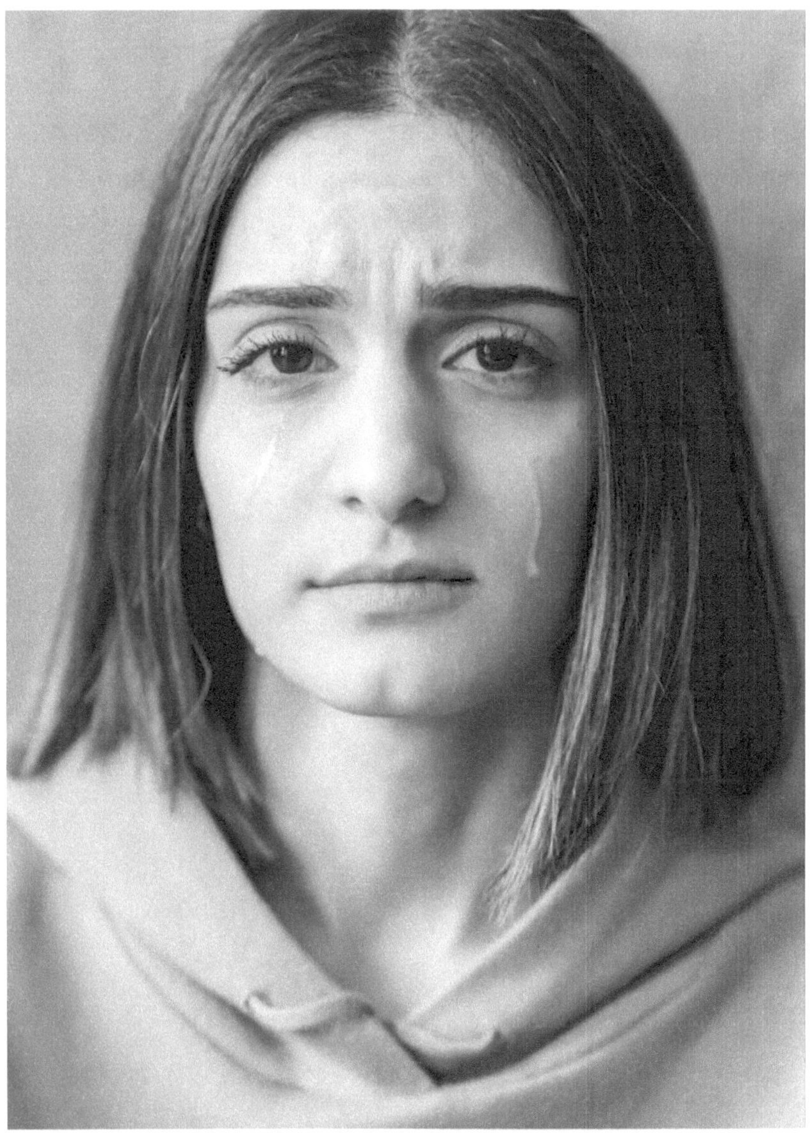

There are so many cases that unfortunately are very common for us to see in the office. It really does suck as both the patient and dental team, yes even the dental team. No one likes to be the bearer of bad news. No one likes to hear bad news, period. But it happens. And I hate to say or even sound like I'm saying I told you so but to be completely transparent, it could all be avoided if you take care of your teeth. I probably sound annoying and maybe even border line lecturing, at the end of the day it is what it is and I'm sharing to help you make a quaint decision to brush like a boss… or not, whichever helps you sleep at night.

11

Protecting your teeth with a couple of do's and don'ts

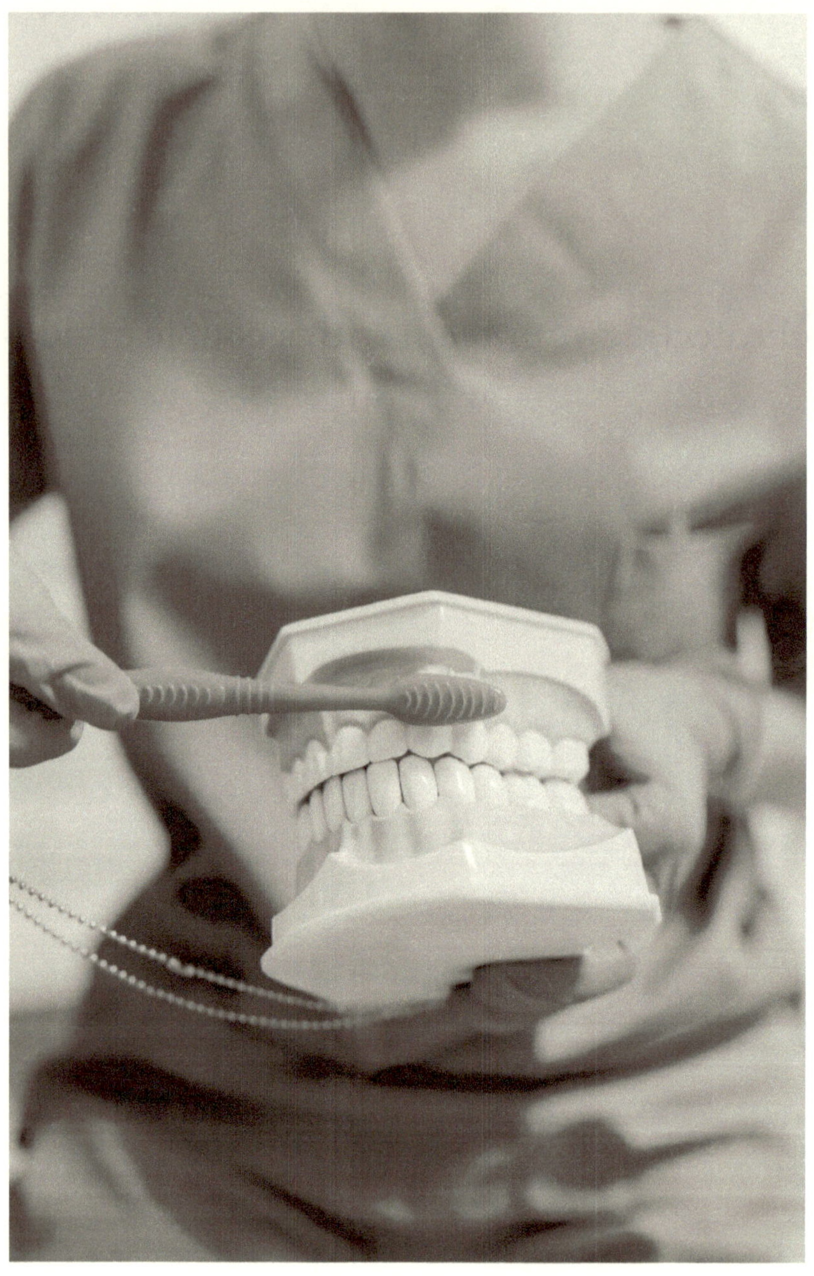

A recap of some of the things that could help protect your teeth while you have them and for the long run!

1. Brush your teeth (sorry not sorry but that is literally the importance of this book)
2. Floss, waterpik and mouthwash is key
3. If you are going to brush once daily, at least do so right before you go to bed. Don't leave those sugar bugs on your teeth even longer than they should stay, they don't deserve a home in your mouth!
4. Food is life! Not going to be a health guru here, because believe me, I'm still working on that part. But the types of food we consume do in fact affect our teeth. Sugary drinks, candies, high carbs, food that stains like spaghetti and even coffee. These may be good for the moment but if not removed off our teeth will cause problems down the road.
5. Mouth guards: night guards, day guards, sports guards for the win! If you are going to focus on anything in life, at least your teeth: your health! If your teeth are perfectly fine, invest in one of these guards! Lots of people don't think they grind their teeth or better yet clench, but ooh wee am I here to tell you there is a vast majority of us who do it and don't even realize we are. Better to do damage to a mouth guard than your own teeth right? Unfortunately, most insurances do not help and feel this is more of a cosmetic thing and I cannot help but disagree, it's a lot to unpack. But if finances allow, please do consider getting one, your teeth will thank you. And once you do, just like anything else, it takes time to get used to wearing one. Do your own research on them, you'll thank me later.

6. Pacifiers (binky's), thumb sucking and even nail biting are some of the worst things we can do to our teeth. Yes, for that time being it definitely helps in that time period but in fact it's doing more harm. Baby teeth are in fact baby teeth and will eventually fall out but the way we care for baby teeth do pave the way for adult teeth to develop. So, the sooner you can kick that habit of reaching for a binky or thumb sucking or even biting your nails, the better chance your teeth have in staying for the long run.

7. Do the best you can. Visit your dentist. Try to make it a habit before the pain persists. If you forget your routine one day, guess what, when you wake up, there's another chance for you to try again. I am not here to be your coach or your cheerleader but for someone who is very passionate and has been in the field for over a decade. I am here to help you try because those teeth you do end up keeping will have done their job. How? Well, how's that new recipe you tried tasting? Your teeth help you chew it up? Your stomach like it? Are you tasting that flavor with every bite? I bet you are. Not trying to throw it in your face, but, seriously you've got this because your teeth depend on it, that simple.

12

Conclusion

Overall, how you care for your teeth will reflect in your everyday health. It is the gateway to all major health concerns. Don't believe me, do your own research. Talk to your dentist, sit in a seminar, do what you have to do to get the answers you need on how or what you have to do to keep your teeth. My only ask is that when you do find the answers you need, take the courage to act on that and care for your teeth. Brush like a boss, you'll feel like one when the dentist tells you how great they look! This was indeed the ultimate guide to caring for the teeth (and gums) you want to keep. I hope it was as thrilling to you to read as it was for me to write.

Respectfully,

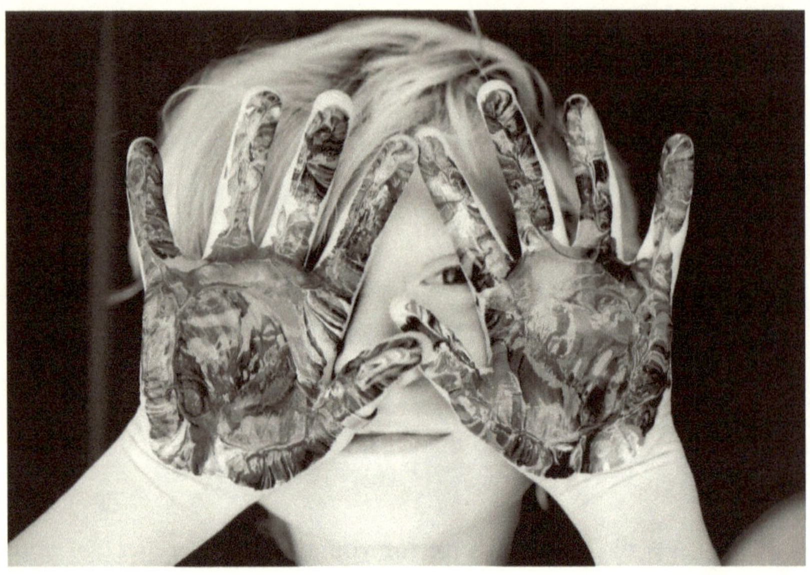

Elizabeth Shelton

Resources:

1. **World Health Organization: WHO. (2019, November 14).** *Oral health.* **https://www.who.int/health-topics/oral-health#tab=tab_1**

1. **World Health Organization: WHO. (2023, March 14).** *Oral health.* **https://www.who.int/news-room/fact-sheets/detail/oral-health**